SEX COUPONS FOR

Her

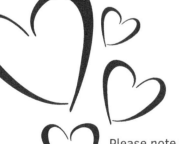

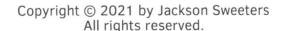

The cover has been designed using resources from Freepik.com
Designed by starline / Freepik

THIS COUPON ENTITLES YOU TO:

HOTEL SEX

TERMS & CONDITIONS: _____

_____

_____

0 123456789 87

THIS COUPON ENTITLES YOU TO:

A HARD RIDE

TERMS & CONDITIONS:

0 123456789 87

THIS COUPON ENTITLES YOU TO:

THE KINKIEST SEX YOU WANT

0 123456789 87

TERMS & CONDITIONS:

_____

_____

_____

THIS COUPON ENTITLES YOU TO:

TIE ME UP

TERMS & CONDITIONS:

_____

_____

_____

0 123456789 87

THIS COUPON ENTITLES YOU TO:

ORAL STIMULATION

0 123456789 87

TERMS & CONDITIONS:

THIS COUPON ENTITLES YOU TO:

A FREE NAUGHTY WISH

0 123456789 87

TERMS & CONDITIONS:

_____

_____

_____

THIS COUPON ENTITLES YOU TO:

QUICKIE

0 123456789 87

TERMS & CONDITIONS:

_____

_____

_____

THIS COUPON ENTITLES YOU TO:

A ROMANTIC SHOWER FOR TWO

TERMS & CONDITIONS:

_____

_____

_____

THIS COUPON ENTITLES YOU TO:

ANAL PLEASURE

0 123456789 87

TERMS & CONDITIONS:

_____

_____

_____

THIS COUPON ENTITLES YOU TO:

NIGHT OF LOVE

0 123456789 87

TERMS & CONDITIONS:

_____

_____

_____

THIS COUPON ENTITLES YOU TO:

A MASSAGE WITH HAPPY ENDING

0 123456789 87

TERMS & CONDITIONS:

THIS COUPON ENTITLES YOU TO:

A YOU-CHOOSE-THE-TOY NIGHT

0 123456789 87

TERMS & CONDITIONS:

_____

_____

_____

THIS COUPON ENTITLES YOU TO:

ROLE PLAYING

TERMS & CONDITIONS:

_____

_____

_____

THIS COUPON ENTITLES YOU TO:

MIDDLE OF NIGHT SEX

TERMS & CONDITIONS:
_____
_____
_____

0 123456789 87

THIS COUPON ENTITLES YOU TO:

A NAUGHTY FOOT RUB

0 123456789 87

TERMS & CONDITIONS:

_____

_____

_____

THIS COUPON ENTITLES YOU TO:

A SECRET DESIRE

0 123456789 87

TERMS & CONDITIONS:

_____

_____

_____

THIS COUPON ENTITLES YOU TO:

PLAY DRESS UP

0 123456789 87

TERMS & CONDITIONS:

_____

_____

_____

THIS COUPON ENTITLES YOU TO:

A PASSIONATE EVENING

0 123456789 87

TERMS & CONDITIONS:
_____

_____

_____

THIS COUPON ENTITLES YOU TO:

USE HANDCUFFS

TERMS & CONDITIONS:

0 123456789 87

THIS COUPON ENTITLES YOU TO:

A LONG FOREPLAY

0 123456789 87

TERMS & CONDITIONS:

_____

_____

_____

THIS COUPON ENTITLES YOU TO:

ONE SEX SESSION, ANYTIME, ANYWHERE

0 123456789 87

TERMS & CONDITIONS:
_____
_____
_____

THIS COUPON ENTITLES YOU TO:

I'LL TAKE ALL MY CLOTHES OFF, WHATEVER I'M DOING

0 123456789 87

TERMS & CONDITIONS:

_____

_____

_____

THIS COUPON ENTITLES YOU TO:

FUN WITH CHOCOLATE BODY PAINT

TERMS & CONDITIONS:

0 123456789 87

THIS COUPON ENTITLES YOU TO:

A ROMANTIC BUBBLE BATH FOR TWO

TERMS & CONDITIONS: _____

_____

_____

0 123456789 87

THIS COUPON ENTITLES YOU TO:

GO SKINNY DIPPING

0 123456789 87

TERMS & CONDITIONS:

_____

_____

_____

THIS COUPON ENTITLES YOU TO:

A NEW SEXY EXPERIMENT

0 123456789 87

TERMS & CONDITIONS:

_____

_____

_____

THIS COUPON ENTITLES YOU TO:

FISTING SESSION

0 123456789 87

TERMS & CONDITIONS:

_____

_____

_____

THIS COUPON ENTITLES YOU TO:

A NEW SURPRISE SEX TOY

0 123456789 87

TERMS & CONDITIONS:

_____

_____

_____

THIS COUPON ENTITLES YOU TO:

PLAYTIME IN JUST TIE AND HEELS

TERMS & CONDITIONS:

0 123456789 87

THIS COUPON ENTITLES YOU TO:

MORNING SEX

0 123456789 87

TERMS & CONDITIONS:

_____

_____

_____

THIS COUPON ENTITLES YOU TO:

ONE NEW POSITION EVERY NIGHT FOR A WEEK

0 123456789 87

TERMS & CONDITIONS:

_____

_____

_____

THIS COUPON ENTITLES YOU TO:

TIE ME UP AND USE BLINDFOLDS

0 123456789 87

TERMS & CONDITIONS: _____

_____

_____

THIS COUPON ENTITLES YOU TO:

15 MINUTES OF PLAYING WITH BALLS

0 123456789 87

TERMS & CONDITIONS:
_____
_____
_____

THIS COUPON ENTITLES YOU TO:

MAKE OUT IN PUBLIC

0 123456789 87

TERMS & CONDITIONS:
_____
_____
_____

THIS COUPON ENTITLES YOU TO:

SEX OUTSIDE

TERMS & CONDITIONS:

_____

_____

_____

0 123456789 87

THIS COUPON ENTITLES YOU TO:

FULL MORNING OF FOREPLAYING

0 123456789 87

TERMS & CONDITIONS:

_____

_____

_____

THIS COUPON ENTITLES YOU TO:

HE-DOES-ALL-THE-WORK SESSION

0 123456789 87

TERMS & CONDITIONS:

_____

_____

_____

THIS COUPON ENTITLES YOU TO:

CREAM BLOWJOBS

0 123456789 87

TERMS & CONDITIONS:
_____
_____
_____

THIS COUPON ENTITLES YOU TO:

AN INTIMATE PICNIC

0 123456789 87

TERMS & CONDITIONS:

_____

_____

_____

THIS COUPON ENTITLES YOU TO:

THREESOME

TERMS & CONDITIONS:

_____

_____

_____

0 123456789 87

THIS COUPON ENTITLES YOU TO:

PORN MOVIE NIGHT

0 123456789 87

TERMS & CONDITIONS:

_____

_____

_____

THIS COUPON ENTITLES YOU TO:

WAKE-UP SEX

0 123456789 87

TERMS & CONDITIONS:

_____

_____

_____

THIS COUPON ENTITLES YOU TO:

YOUR DESIRED LINE OF DIRTY TALK DURING SEX

0 123456789 87

TERMS & CONDITIONS:

_____

_____

_____

THIS COUPON ENTITLES YOU TO:

COWGIRL SESSION

0 123456789 87

TERMS & CONDITIONS:

_____

_____

_____

THIS COUPON ENTITLES YOU TO:

SIXTY-NINE

0 123456789 87

TERMS & CONDITIONS:

_____

_____

_____

THIS COUPON ENTITLES YOU TO:

RIDE ME HARD

TERMS & CONDITIONS:
_____

_____

_____

0 123456789 87

THIS COUPON ENTITLES YOU TO:

ONE SPANKING SESSION

0 123456789 87

TERMS & CONDITIONS:

_____

_____

_____

THIS COUPON ENTITLES YOU TO:

TAKE FULL CONTROL DURING SEX

TERMS & CONDITIONS:
_____

_____

_____

0 123456789 87

THIS COUPON ENTITLES YOU TO:

ONE MUTUAL MASTURBATION SESSION

TERMS & CONDITIONS:

0 123456789 87

THIS COUPON ENTITLES YOU TO:

A NIGHT WITH BLINDFOLDS

TERMS & CONDITIONS: _____
_____
_____

0 123456789 87

THIS COUPON ENTITLES YOU TO:

0 123456789 87

TERMS & CONDITIONS:

THIS COUPON ENTITLES YOU TO:

0 123456789 87

TERMS & CONDITIONS:

THIS COUPON ENTITLES YOU TO:

0 123456789 87

TERMS & CONDITIONS:

THIS COUPON ENTITLES YOU TO:

0 123456789 87

TERMS & CONDITIONS:

THIS COUPON ENTITLES YOU TO:

_____

0 123456789 87

TERMS & CONDITIONS:

_____

_____

_____

THIS COUPON ENTITLES YOU TO:

TERMS & CONDITIONS:

0 123456789 87

THIS COUPON ENTITLES YOU TO:

0 123456789 87

TERMS & CONDITIONS:

THIS COUPON ENTITLES YOU TO:

0 123456789 87

TERMS & CONDITIONS:

THIS COUPON ENTITLES YOU TO:

0 123456789 87

TERMS & CONDITIONS:

THIS COUPON ENTITLES YOU TO:

0 123456789 87

TERMS & CONDITIONS:

THANK YOU!

Thanks for buying *Sex Coupons For Her*.

If your found the book funny and enjoyed your time using the coupons, please share your thoughts about it on Amazon by leaving a review.

Also, if you want to discover more amazing books by Jackson Sweeters, check out his author page from Amazon. Just search "Jackson Sweeters" on Amazon's search bar and you'll find it.

Made in the USA
Monee, IL
31 December 2024